Computers and Your Health

Protecting yourself from Computer Related Health Issues

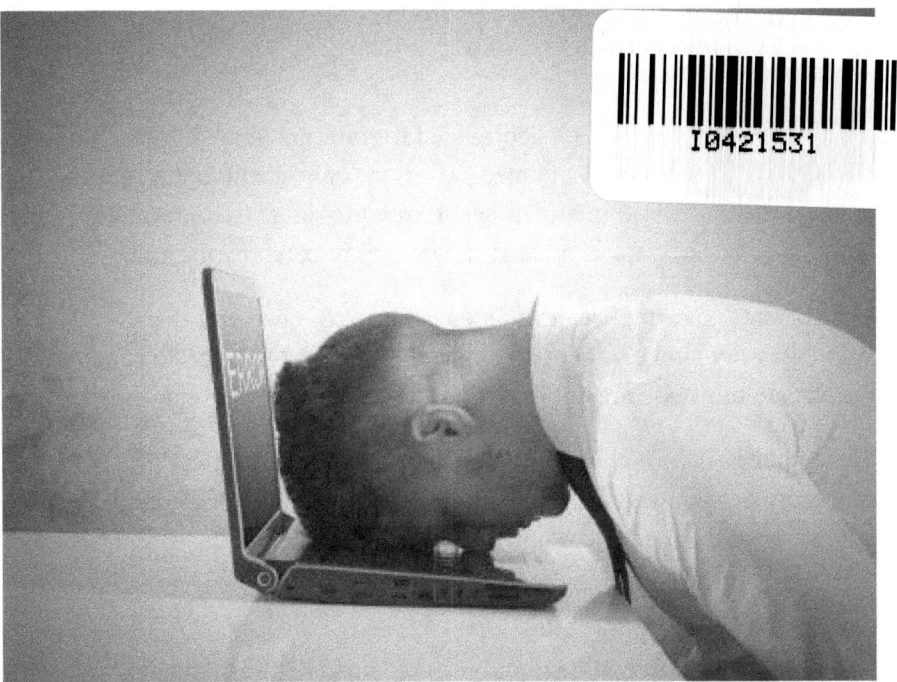

Dueep Jyot Singh

Mendon Cottage Books

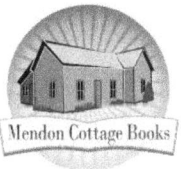

JD-Biz Publishing

Our books are available at

1. Amazon.com

2. Barnes and Noble

3. Itunes

4. Kobo

5. Smashwords

6. Google Play Books

Table of Contents

Introduction

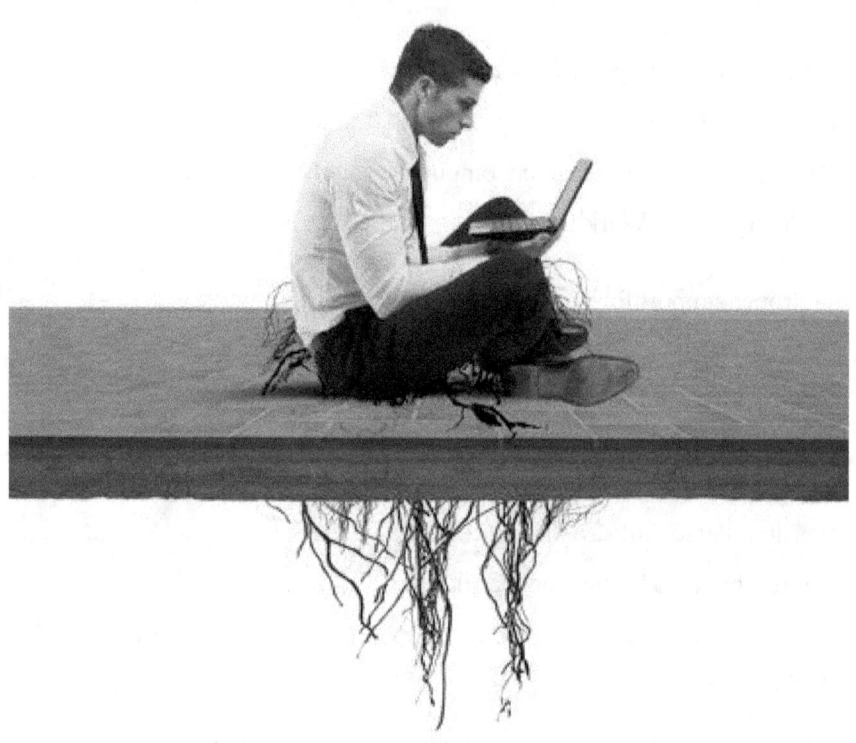

So, all right, getting addicted to computers and thus growing roots, sitting in one place may sound and look hilarious, but computer addiction and computer abuse is one of the main concerns of the 21st century.

This is going to occur when you use computers at a stretch. Consider this to be a hydra which is going to affect your body, state of mind and your lifestyle.

Once upon the time, we welcomed 21st-century technology in our lives with open arms, because we thought it would make our lives easier with the advent of the World Wide Web, computers have become a center of attention, and an integral part of our lives.

Despite all the problems computers give us, including general security faults, crashing when you have a deadline to meet, and other constant reminders that they are only as good as the people who use them, man has stepped into an entirely new culture and lifestyle revolving around computers and other Internet-based machines.

This book is going to introduce you to the concept of computer abuse and how it is going to affect your health as well as your social life. But before that, you need to ask yourself how many times you have checked your email today? How many hours of the day do you spend getting in touch with your friends on social networking sites? Do you spend a major part of the day browsing for Internet sites where you can get information about the subjects of your interest?

And last but not the least, have you found yourself neglecting your family, friends, and other people in your social circle, just because you could not be pulled away from your computer.

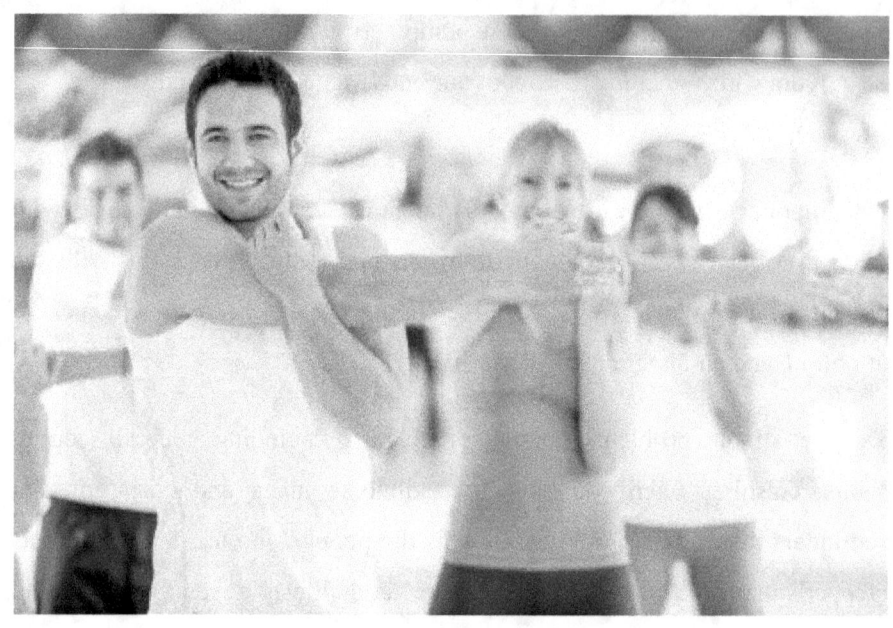

No computers for the next hour…

You are a fairly good example of a future computer addict. This addiction is definitely not restricted to a computer. It is also seen all over the world in the form of cell phone addiction and tablet addiction where the first thing you do when you wake up is check the messages on your smart phone and see who has sent you a message during the far reaches of the night when he was suffering from insomnia.

This is something which you are going to repeat last thing at night, before you switch your phone off. It is going to beep throughout the night, sending you messages from your friends, colleagues, RSS feeds, breaking news, Tickertape headlines, and so on.

Spending anywhere over 6 hours a day at the computer, for even as little as a year, can cause a plethora of computer related problems and disorders.

This book is going to tell you all about practical remedies for these self-induced problems, and how you can manage to prevent them from taking over your life.

The Hazard of Eyestrain

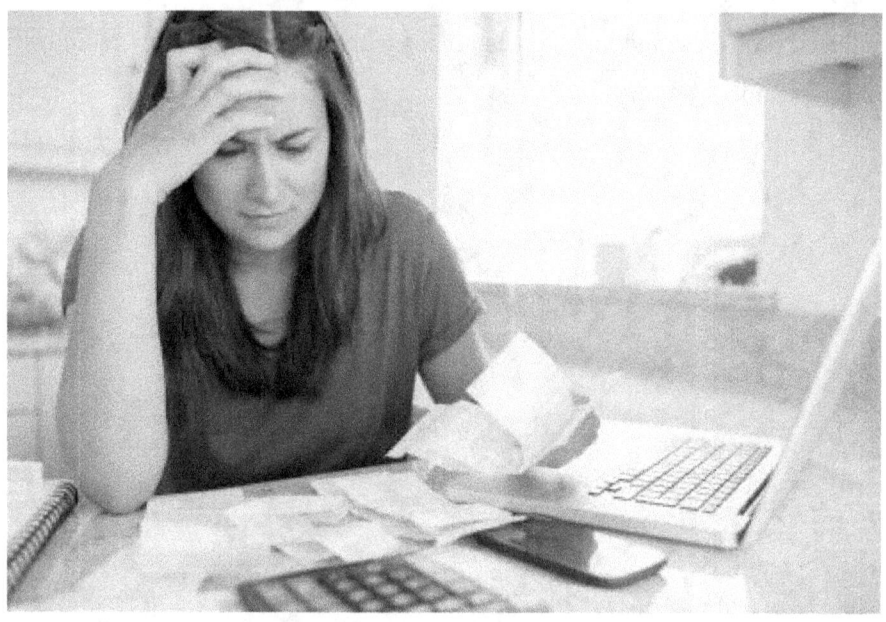

Bills, bills, bills, and eyestrain. As if I did not have headaches enough...

One of the occupational hazards of sitting in front of the computer is computer strain and eyestrain. For many of us, this is a part and parcel of our lives, because working on a computer is job related. On the other hand, you should not be surprised to see youngsters with ophthalmologic refractive errors increasing, just because they spend most of their time either in chat rooms, or talking to their friends, or just playing games on the Internet.

There are so many people in the world today, who are suffering from these problems. You can consider this to be a Surfeit of Computers, with apologies to the Bard.

Such compulsive users of the Internet are definitely going to be suffering from eyestrain in the future, if they have not begun to suffer from it right now. This is going to take the form of red eyes, mild headaches and also possible spondylitis along with accompanying side effect pain in the neck and in the lower back. And because modern technology makes it necessary for a large percentage of youngsters and school children to sit continuously before a screen, is it surprising that the strain is felt in the eyes before it is felt in the rest of the body.

This is because the eyes are being subject to some sort of trauma without any let up. This is going to manifest itself in the form of eyestrain, blurred vision, dry and irritated eyes, and headaches.

The biggest difference between adults and children experience symptoms is that children do not know when to stop. Unless they are disciplined, and a check is kept on their activities, they are going to continue playing on the computers. Adults have common sense and they know when to switch off the computer. Even then, there are a number of us who decide that we are going to switch off the computer in 10 minutes and we just need to complete this bit of work, and the 10 minute stretch on and on.

If this can happen to us, how can we blame children, especially when their eyes are literally streaming with tears and crying for mercy. Kids do not think of taking a break, especially when they are doing something which interests them. They also do not know anything about the screen contrast.

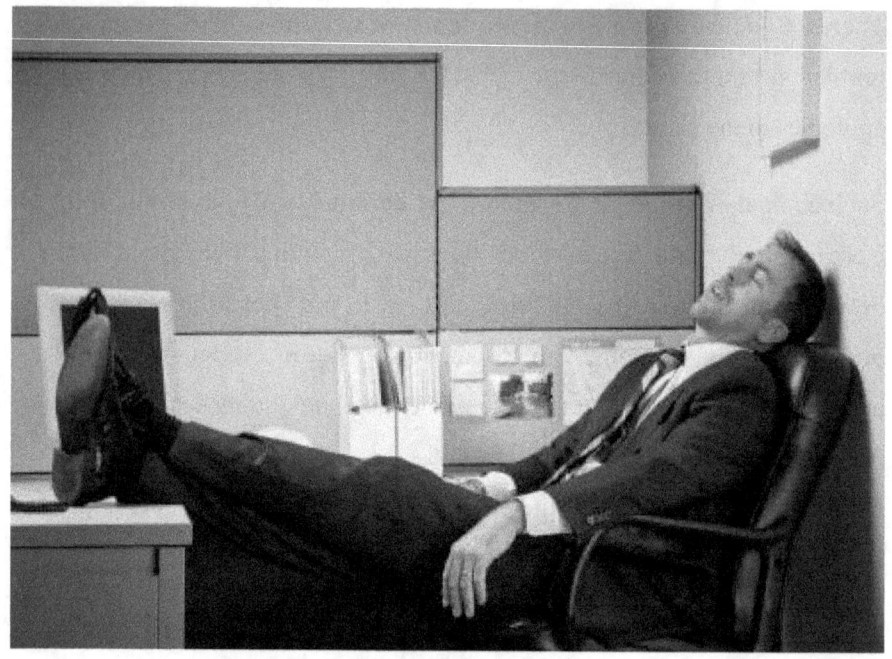

They also do not know how the height of a computer can make all the difference between pain in the neck and an enjoyable computer session. They are just going to continue to work on the computer at the setting preferred by mom or dad.

Eyestrain does not indicate that computer use is causing any damage to your eyes. But this is symptomatic of another potential problem. This means that it is possible that you may be suffering from a possible eye ailment and you need to get prescription glasses.

Minimizing Eyestrain

To make sure that you do not suffer from eyestrain, or to minimize its effect on your general health, try these easy to utilize tips –

1. Set a time limit on continuous usage of computers. A 10 minute break each hour is going to help your body to recover from sitting in one position for a long time without many of the muscles moving.

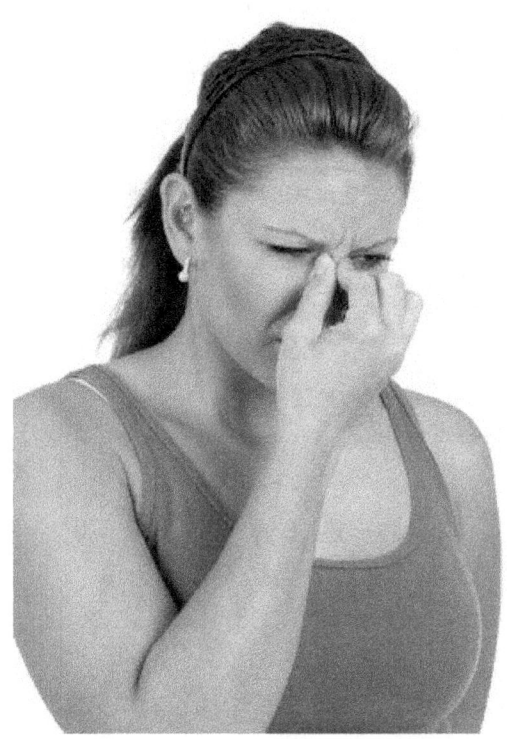

2. Adjust the height of the computer screen. Children should view the screen at a 15° downward angle. It should be 4 – 9 inches below the eye level. The screen should be 24 – 26 inches away from the eyes. This means that they will not be required to tilt their head in a downward position or tense their neck muscles.

3. The lighting should be adjusted in the screen, so that you do not suffer from glare.

4. Here is one Tip which I do whenever I sit in front of a computer, especially one with a blurry screen. [Yes, there are still some non-LCD screens floating around in many parts of the globe, and they "blur" or jump.] These jumpy screens are quite capable of giving you a headache.

Go to the display properties of your desktop and click Settings.

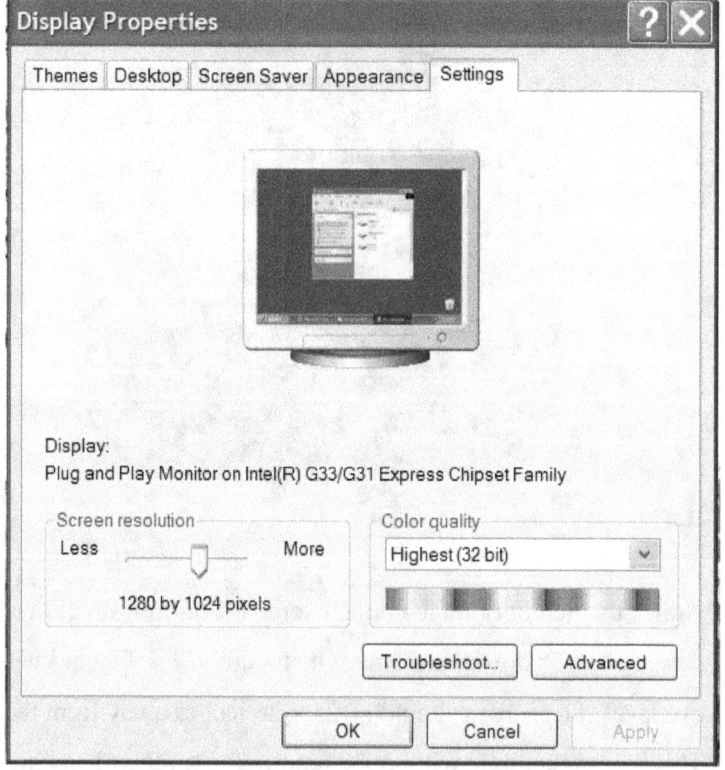

After that, click "Advanced." You are going to be taken to this page below.

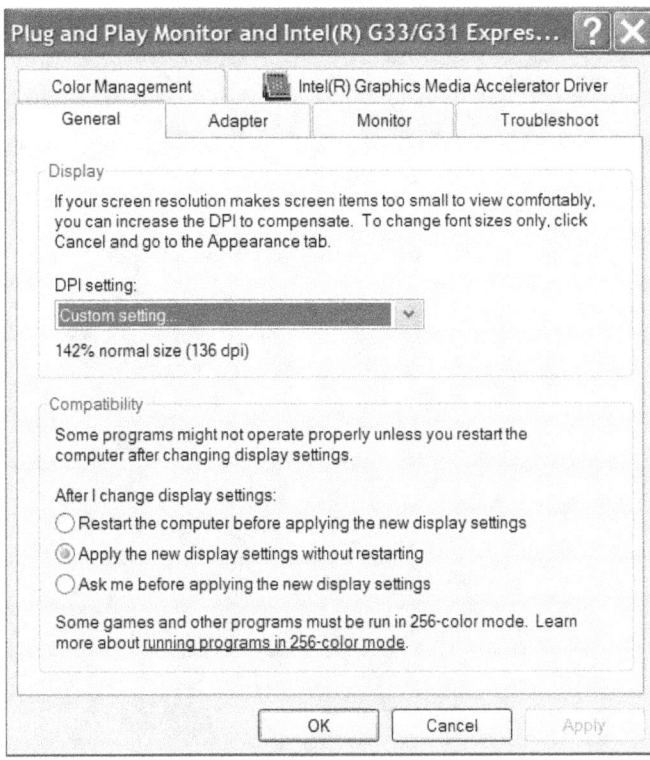

I have customized my personal likes in custom settings, as I want. At the moment, I am interested in the Monitor, next to the Adapter on the navigation bar.

Depending on your requirements, you can change the screen refresh rate from 60 Hertz to 75 Hertz.

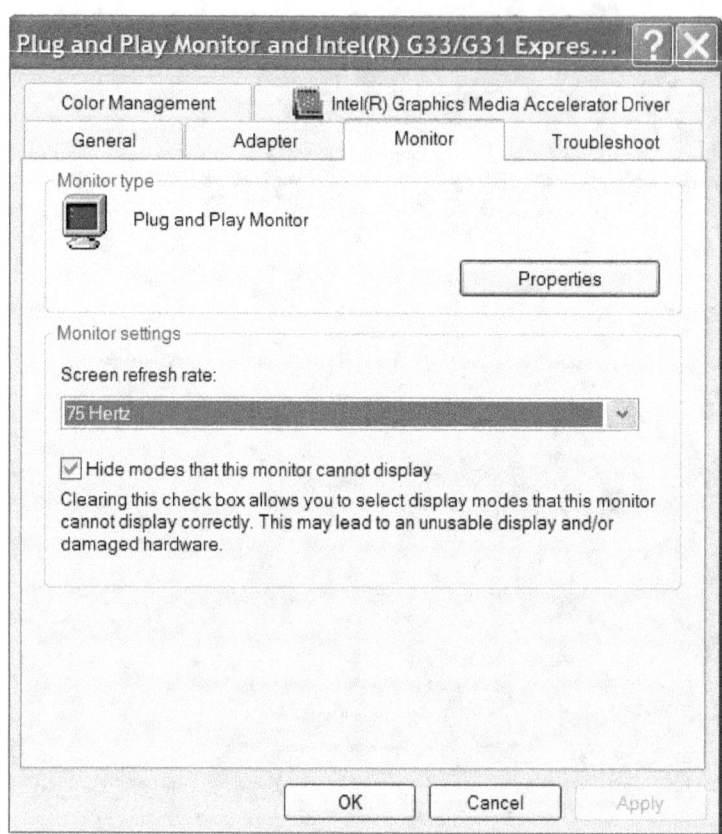

Click okay, and see if you find the screen clearer or not. It is possible that you may find this refresh rate, much to your liking, especially when you find yourself working on the computer for a longer period of time.

Encourage children to blink. When we stare at the screen, continuously, our tear ducts are going to dry up, especially if we keep staring at the screen for a long time without blinking like goggled eyed goldfish. So blinking is going to prevent your eyes from going dry.

Reputed Optometric Associations in the USA have identified 4 characteristics of children which make them more sensitive to vision problems while they are sitting in front of the computer.

These include a limited self-awareness, more adaptability, smaller size than adults and usage of computer in less than ideal lighting conditions. This makes them more vulnerable to eyestrain.

Here are some more computer related problems including carpal syndrome.

Repetitive Strain Injury

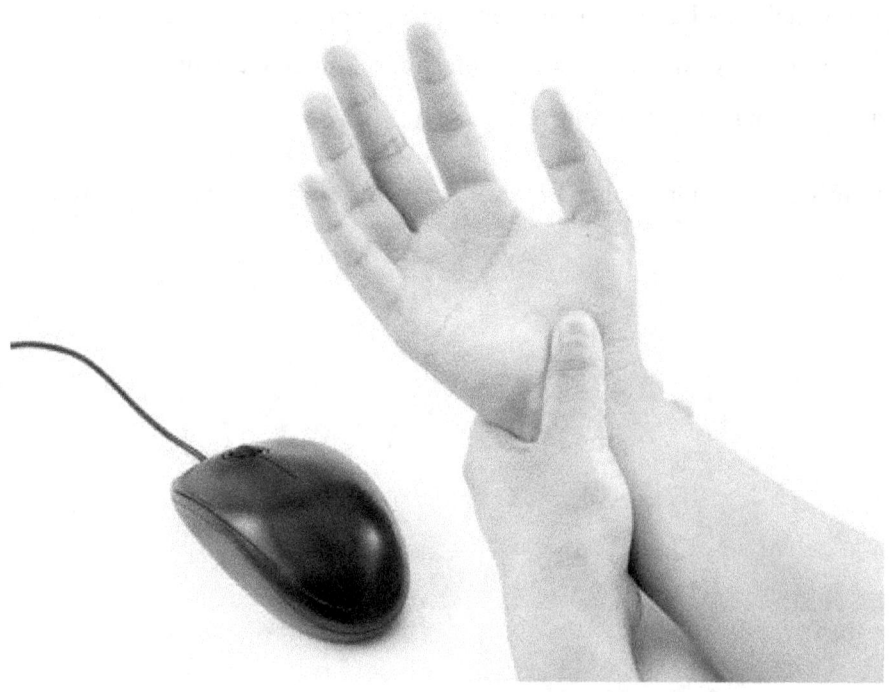

Why are so many youngsters in their teens complaining of pain in the neck and back and wrist problems? Have you heard a youngster say, "Why does my wrist pain so much? This normally occurs after a computer class or after I have had a session on the computer. And sometimes, I feel these shooting pains, apropos of nothing. Oh dear, what can the matter be?[1]"

---

[1] The last line can be disregarded. Hear any teenager saying this. He is going to be hooted and booted out of his peers' circle as being a sissy.

This is an injury due to a prolonged use of the computer mouse. This is Repetitive Strain Injury [RSI.] This is one of the most prevalent diseases found in frequent computer users. This is the term used to describe pain, injuries, or disfiguration of any upper extremity due to the overuse of certain tendons and muscles.

Most of the people suffering from RSI are in the 18 – 24 year old age group. 60% of them are going to suffer from neck and back pain. 25% are going to complain of pain in hands and wrists. 6% are going to suffer from pain in the lower limbs and back.

Once upon a time, patients over the age of 50 found themselves suffering from cervical and lumbar spondylitis, but sadly enough, now even teenagers are beginning to complain of these symptoms. This is due to excessive computer use. That is because your neck is in one stiff position for a long period of time and the muscles do not get a chance to exercise themselves much.

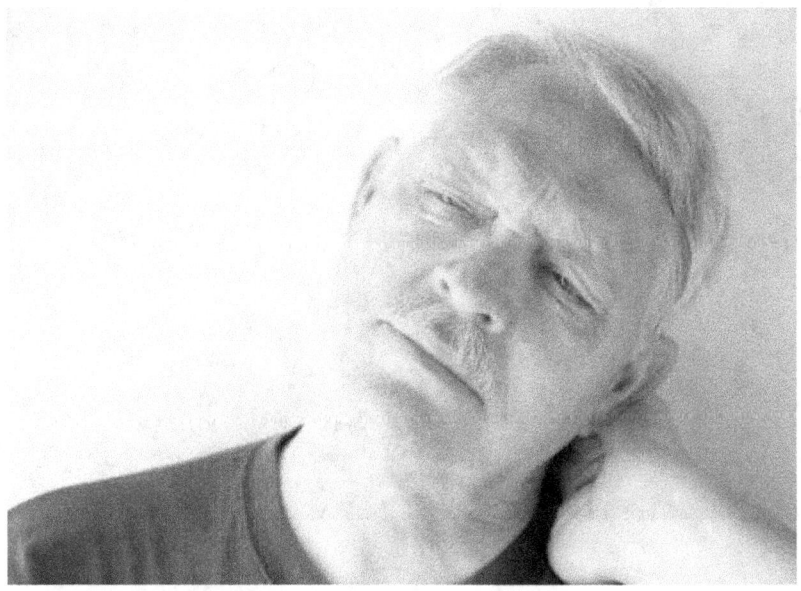

More than 80% of the computer users are going to suffer from some kind of physical problem. This is related to the increased usage of a mouse.

A mouse is going to sit on the side of the keyboard. You must reach out to use it. That means you are going to put twice as much strain on your neck, shoulder and arm muscles, when compared to the amount of strain utilized when you are using a track ball or a pointed device mounted in the center of the keyboard.

This last facility is of course is not available on our modern-day keyboards. We keep following the mouse.

Carpal Tunnel Syndrome

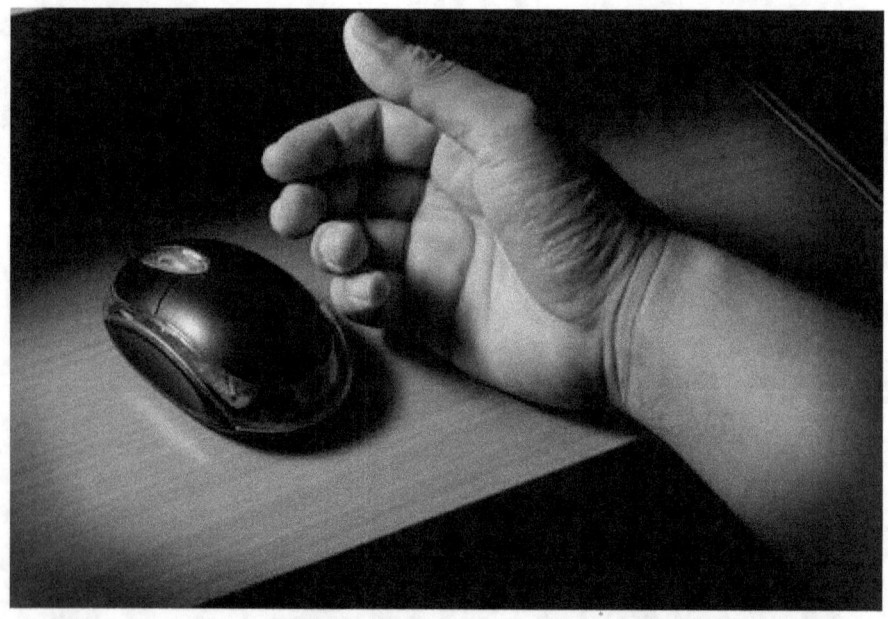

Any muscle, which has been has been held tense at even 18% of its maximum effort is going to reduce the blood flow through the tissues by 80%. This is research data taken from the Journal of ergonomics, published somewhere around 2003. It is, of course, still valid today.

The tight muscles, which result from continuous smalls usage is also going to pinch nerves. This is also going to cause pain down into the hands and the wrists. That means you are suffering from carpal to nose syndrome, which is a painful and debilitating condition.

This problem involves the flexor tendons, and the median nerve that extends from the forearm into your hand. These are going to extend through a tunnel, which is made up off the wrist bones and the transverse carpal ligament.

As you move your fingers and your hands, the flexor tendons are going to rub against the side of the tunnel. This rubbing can cause irritation of the tendons. This is going to cause them to swell. When the tendons swell, they are going to apply pressure upon the median nerve.

This result is going to be either a tingling sensation, numbness and then possible pain and eventual disability.

Computer users are not the only ones suffering from carpal tendon syndrome. Musicians as well as artisans using their hands extensively also suffer from this ailment.

Children and Computer Related Problems

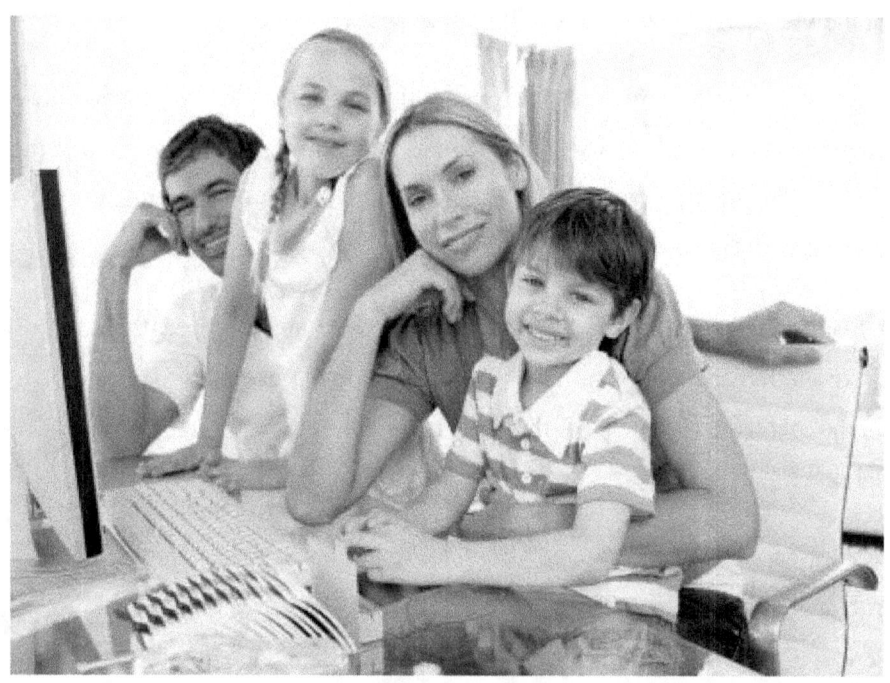

We intend to teach our children how to use computers safely.

Children are more prone to problems appearing from prolonged usage of computers. That is because they are particularly at risk because their muscles and bones are still in the development phase and growing stage.

Ergonomic experts have found out that millions of youngsters are using equipment which was initially designed for adults, both at school and at home. These children are using the computers which were initially set up for adults.

That is why they are more at risk of developing permanent and painful injuries.

Have you noticed that computer keyboards, the mouse, and computer furniture rarely takes into account the diminutive size of children?

Most parents would not, for example, put an 8 year old on an adult sized cycle, and then tell him, "Okay then, you are on your own, learn how to cycle on this monstrosity." They start them out on kids sized cycles.

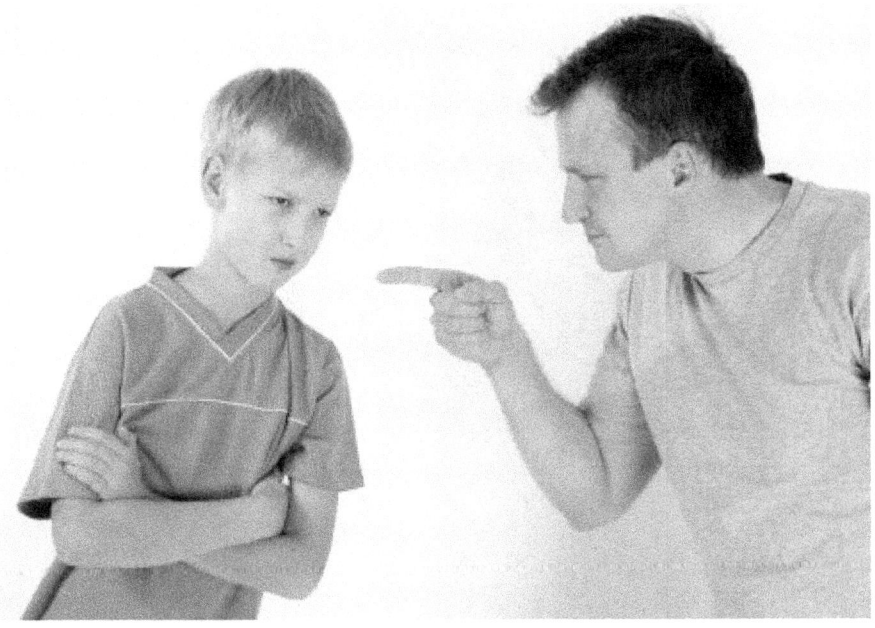

If I see you wasting your time on that downloaded speedster game again...

However, they do not bother much about the possible dangers of children sitting for long periods in front of a computer and in one position, with their wrists over – extended and their necks twisted.

This meant that they had begun on the road to potential back pain, as kids. And they were going to be the future workforce, with one ailment already in place – back pain and a possibly deformed musculature.

Therefore, there is need to develop more user-friendly equipment for children, especially in the matters of computers. Also more research has to be carried out to find the health hazards of excessive usage of the computers on the physical growth of children.

You as a parent need to monitor their computer usage at home, making sure that they take regular breaks. Teach them to sit properly.

Preventing RSI

Get the best computer furniture. Use chairs with the back and neck support. The height of your seat and the positioning of your backrest should be adjustable.

If you have a chair on wheels, there is nothing like it. That means you can change your position by just wheeling your chair in another direction. An armrest on your chair is often helpful to relax your elbows.

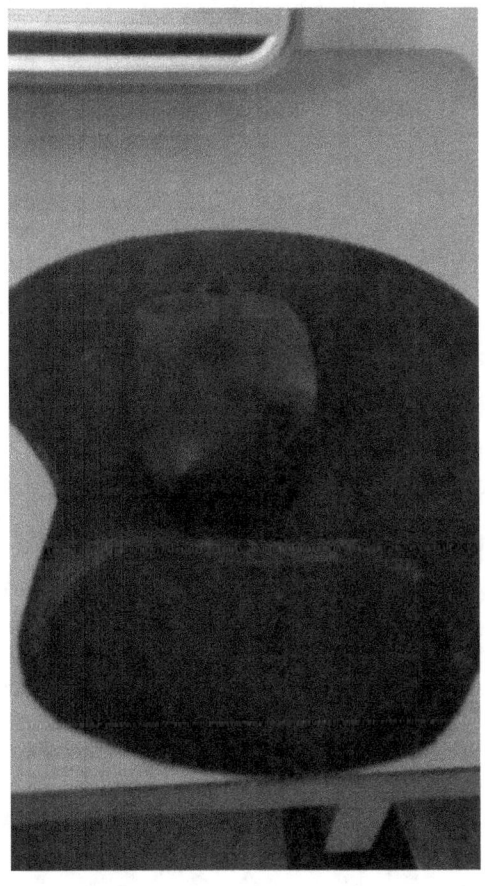

A good way to relax your wrist and give it support is to have a mouse pad with a raised wrist support pad. That means you can continue using your mouse over a longer period of time without bothering much about wrist pain.

Also, cord less mice are a much better idea because you can sit far away from your computer and do the navigation on your desktop with the mouse placed in a comfortable position near your chair.

The table height should be around 27 – 29 inches above the floor. Tall people usually prefer slightly higher tables. Ergonomic computer furniture designs are coming up with ideas will you as a computer user will not be allowed to sit. You will need to do all the work on the computer, standing up or leaning against a support.

I think this idea is a flop show, because half of the fun of sitting in front of the computer is the opportunity to put your feet up and relax.

If you can adjust your table, then set the angle of your waist at 90° and see that your elbow makes a 90° angle when your hands are on the keyboard.

With the elbows and the earliest at 90° angle, your feet are going to rest comfortably flat on the floor. If you do not have an adjustable table, you can try using a raised footrest in order to keep your blood circulation moving well in your lower extremities, and preventing your feet from swelling up.

Repercussions of Extensive Computer Usage

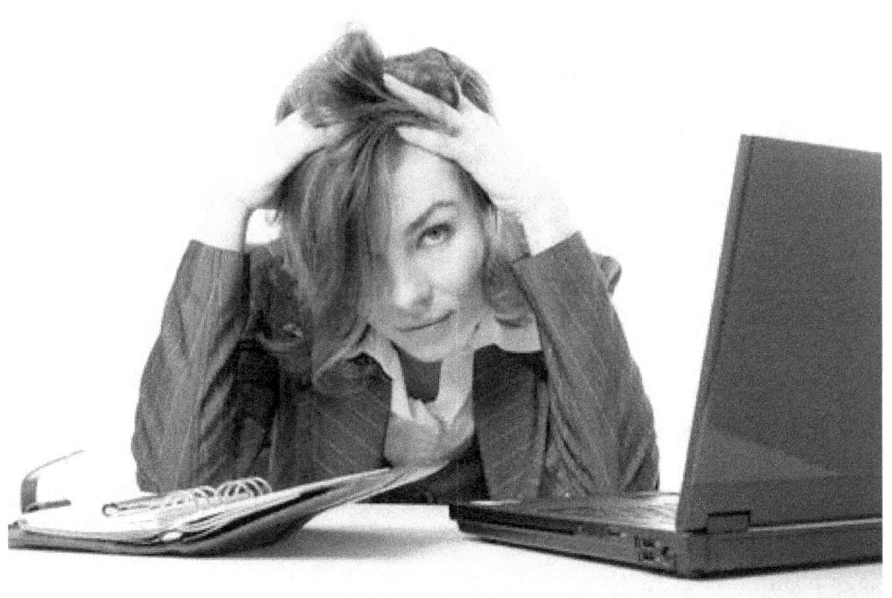

I normally sit anywhere between 7 to 9 hours in front of the desktop computer. After that, I just pick up my tablet and stretched out on my bed, spend another 2 hours or more, browsing on the Internet, watching movies, listening to music, or doing whatever comes to mind, in my own way of relaxing and unwinding after a day's hard work. This makes me a confirmed computer /screen machine addict.

That is of course, in between checking my smart phone for messages, email, updates or any other necessary information sent to me by friends, colleagues, utility service providers and so on.

So what are the repercussions of such a continued sitting, especially when you are not exercising many parts of the body? Apart from a bad posture, which includes rounded shoulders, neck ache, and weight gain around the tummy, one can consider me to be totally antisocial!

This also means, that the previously physically active life has now become a sedentary lifestyle.

In fact my brother coined the sarcastic term "Cellphish" for all those people who spend all their time glued to a cell phone, when in public, and when they should be supposedly communicating with the people around them.

If you are working in an office, where your boss is one of the 20,000 direct descendants of Genghis Khan[2] and frowns heavily on anybody shifting or moving from his computer console, during office hours, try to stand up at least once, every 20 – 30 minutes just to stretch your neck and get your rib cage position back to normal.

You can also try micro-breaks. That means you are going to stop work for a second or less, every 2 minutes or so. Drop your shoulders to let the tension and stiffness seep out.

Change Your Work Routine

I told you that I spend a number of lots in front of the computer screen every day, including Sundays. But I remember to get up every half an hour to

---

[2] This is a fact, and someone, somewhere decided to count them a couple of years ago. All these people have been found all over the areas conquered by the great Khan, born of his alliances/liaisons with the local populace.

stretch my muscles, stretch my neck, and walk around a bit and possibly get some fresh air or a drink of water.

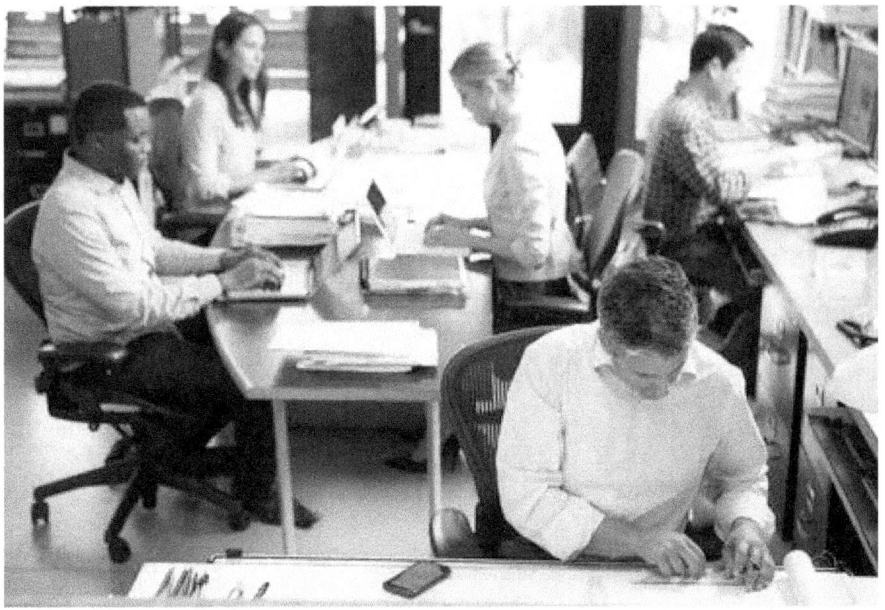

Make sure your daily tasks are not monotonous and repetitive.

This is going to prevent my stomach from staying crunched up in a hunched position. Look at the way you are sitting in front of the computer. Is your chest area stretched, so that you can get a full supply of necessary oxygen into your lungs? Or are you hunched up just like a turtle with your shoulders and the upper portion of your torso, touching your stomach and lower portion of the abdomen with your rib cage all folded up?

Believe it or not, most of us sit in this position because, hey, we are not Victorian, and we never were taught to sit up straight with our spines erect, when we were children.

So even as adults, we are going to sit with our spines and our stomachs in crunched up positions.

Proper support for your neck And Back

What is to stop you from using the neck support pillow, you use when you are traveling in your car, to support your neck when you are sitting in front of the computer?

I bought a number of these neck supports from eBay at really throwaway prices. Some cars, especially the latest models have these included in the seat accessories.

Look for bargains where you can get free international shipping, especially when you get them from Hong Kong, at prices starting from one cent, plus free shipping.

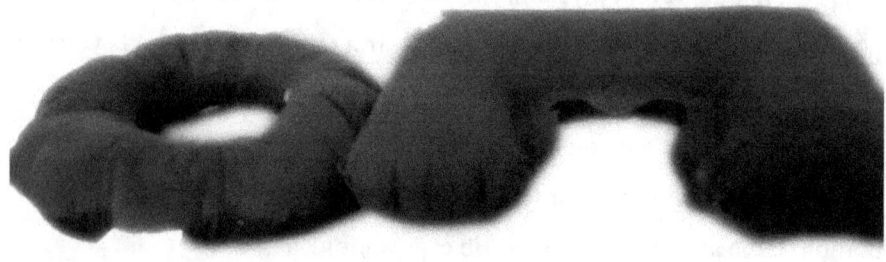

The circular pillow is made up of micro beads, and is excellent for molding itself to the shape of your lower back and neck. The "triangular" pillow is of course an air pillow, but even then, it is very comfortable.

High-Back Chairs

It was somewhere in 2009, when I decided that I needed to get a really good comfortable made-to-measure chair for my computer table.

What is with the high back, made up of a solid plank of wood? Apart from the back support, given to me by a huge cushion, I can just lean back the back of my head on that wood and relax.

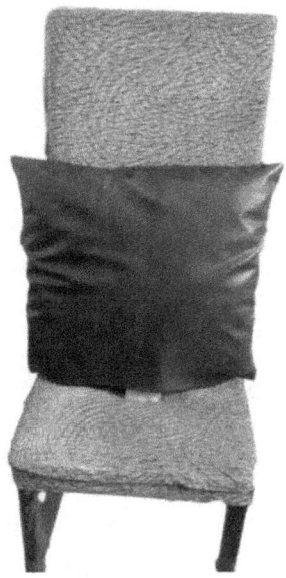

Back dimensions, 27 X 18 inches.

Height of chair – 20 inches from ground, including 2 ½ inches thick Seating.

Seat length and width -20x 21 inches

Of course, this custom-built one-of-a-kind chair design cost me about $20 in material, labor, and fabric, but it has lasted more than 6 years, and it is going to last for another 20 years or so. People going in for looks are going to say Baah, in a Scrooge like tone, but I am more interested in the utility of such a design.

The seat is not made up of cushions. It is a wooden plank on which I can place a cushion, if I want. I can remove the leather covered back support cushion, if I want my back, neck and head supported by the wooden plank back.

So, thanks to such a comfortable and roomy chair/cushions, is it surprising that I am a complete computer-holic?

Practice dynamic sitting, which means keep moving. Do not stay in one position for too long. Also, do not expend too much force punching the keys on your keyboard. Touchpads are such a help in smartphones and tablets, try using them on your desktop PCs or on laptop, if available.

Make sure that your work is not monotonous. Vary your activities throughout the day. This means that you are going to avoid sitting in one position for a number of hours or performing the same action, and hand motion without any interruptions.

You may also want to place the monitor at the right, a reading distance from you. Make sure, the screen is placed in such a way that the content is at eye level. This means that you do not have to lower your head, or raise it in order to read the content.

Keep your keyboard and mouse on a tray so you do not have to reach up to them. They should be tilted away from you, slightly so that can avoid bending your wrists upwards.

Other preventive efforts which are helpful include rotating your usual job for activities which not only demand a change of place and position, but also ask for a change of physical motions, thus setting another set of muscles into play.

Many offices have ergonomically sound workstations, but until you can get your boss or management to set them up for you, you can prevent damage to your body through stretch breaks and other useful and time-tested tips and techniques given above.

RSI Warning Signs

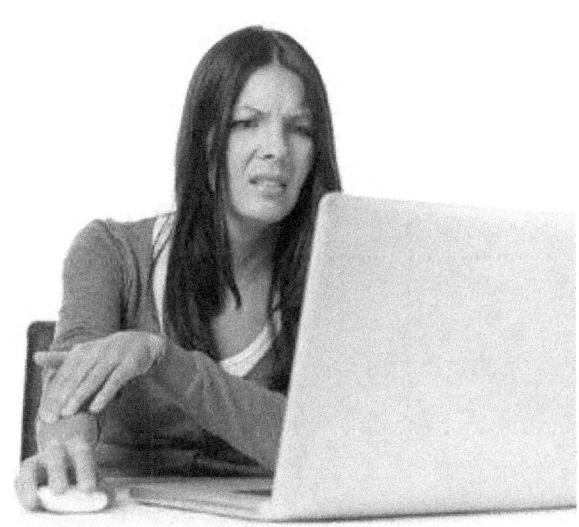

Many parents know all about repetitive stress injury, yet how many of us have bothered to tell our children about this painful condition? So if you or your child is suffering from any sort of tingling sensation in the hand or the wrist, a heaviness or a soreness of your neck, shoulder, upper arms, upper back, elbows, wrists, forearms, fingers and thumbs, it is possible that your muscles and your nerves are on their way to getting stressed out.

In fact, look for these symptoms in yourself or in your child. Do you find yourself massaging a part of your body excessively, or unconsciously? Have you found yourself with a weakening grip in your hand, which may be a forerunner of muscular weakness?

You may also find yourself using your non-dominant hand, to do routine tasks, because using your dominant hand is so painful or uncomfortable.

So how best are you going to cure yourself of this problem? Seek the advice of your health service provider immediately. You do not want extremely painful wrists and swollen hands in the future, do you?

Possible Personality Disorders

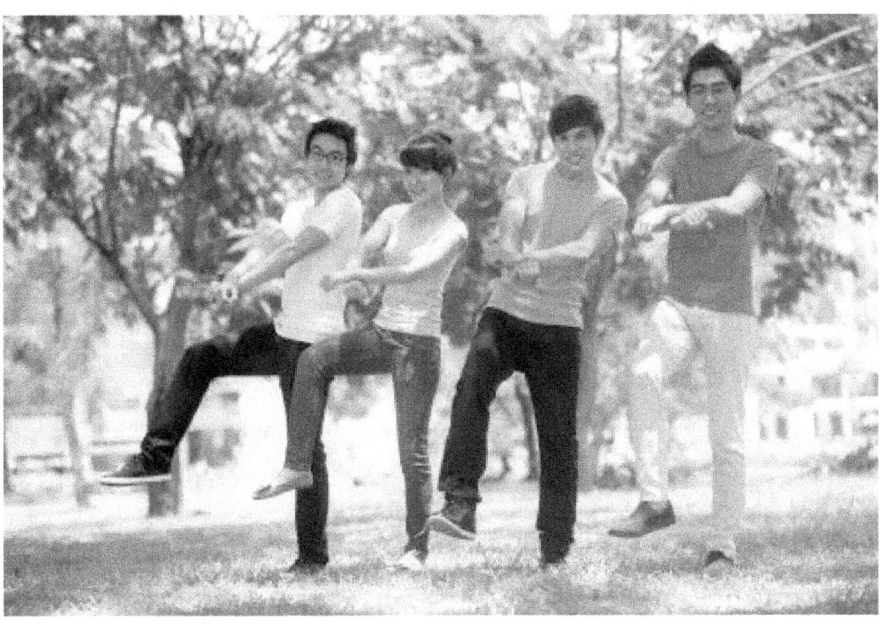

So now here I am, ready to discuss the psychological aspect of excessive computer usage and its effect on our health, and minds as well as personality. Researchers have already begun to tell people that continual, and excessive dependence on computers, smart phones, cell phones, tablets, and so on is getting to be on the rise.

In fact, the traffic officers in our city are really glad, because they have been given permission by the higher authorities to catch hold of anybody using a cell phone while driving. You and I know that this is a totally stupid activity, but believe it or not, there are a number of us, who cannot resist picking up our cell phones while we are driving, and saying, hello while navigating through rush-hour traffic.

We could not be bothered to park our cars on the side of the road and complete our call. We definitely would not ignore the call, and ringing the person back up after we have reached our destination. And of course, we are never going to switch off our phones before we switch on the ignition. And also, because we are human, we have to answer the call right away, forgetting about eyes in front and both hands on steering wheel.

So thanks to this compulsive addiction to computers, as well as other gadgets, is it surprising that about 90% of us are total addicts, even if we do not know it. Many of us, who were social, outgoing and gregarious extroverts can all be found glued to computer/tablets/smart phone screens.

In fact, we have begun to use the computer as a social substitute for human interaction. We would rather make friends online and spend our time and energy chatting with them, instead of talking to our flesh and blood neighbors and friends.

In fact, this was somewhere around 2004, when my then boss got us – faculty, administration and trainee Students [250, in one batch] for a get together. We management, administration and faculty were all asked to place our cell phones outside the get together room, because he did not want to be interrupted with cell phone calls and we of course would never switch off our phones.

The get-together started, and we had just begun to enjoy ourselves, when we found ourselves interrupted by cell phone calls to the students! They just kept excusing themselves with "so sorry, ma'am, sir," and turning away to take the call, until he requested all of them to place their cell phones outside the hall under the close supervision of the security guards.

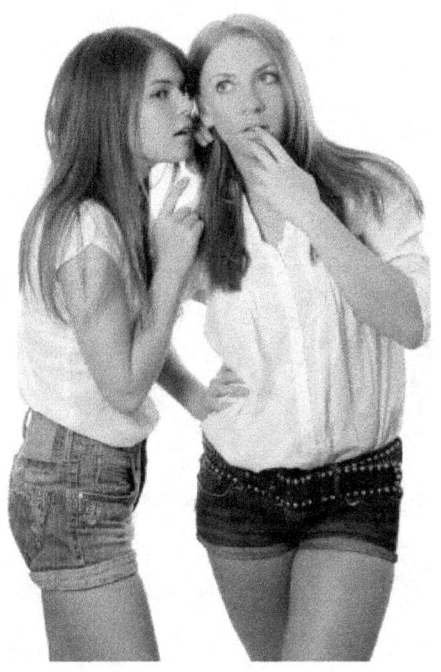

We faculty members/administration were astonished to see 224 cell phones belonging to 250 students, lined up.[3] Nearly all of them were the latest models, making us elders look a bit askance and possibly envious at our old, but tested and true phones.

This was in 2004, and today, nearly every person who can afford a smart phone is going to get one. In fact, my 12 year old nephew passed on his old

---

[3] Yes, we counted them. We are human, are not we?

model to his 7-year-old sister, when he managed to persuade his father to buy him the latest model. She was definitely not amused!

I am not discussing the psychological need for the latest status symbol. Instead, I am worried about our dependence on these objects in order to project our need to fit in with the crowd.

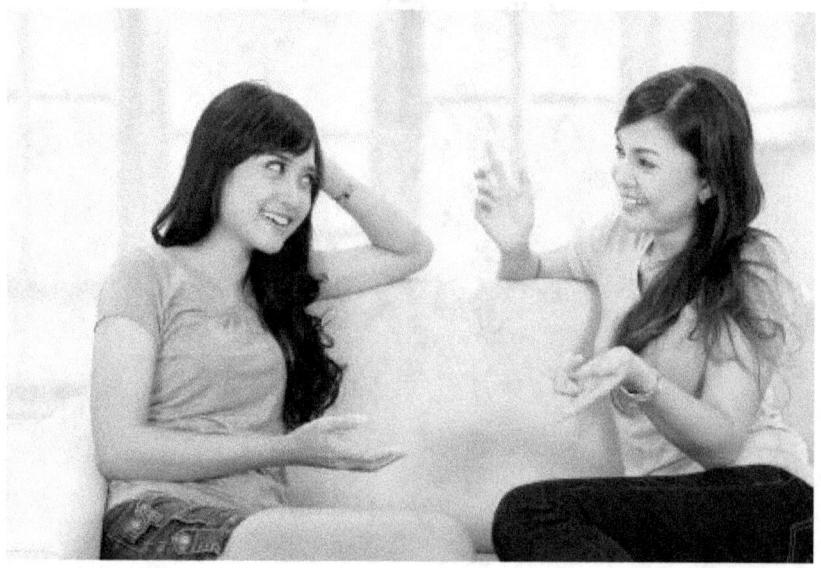

Also, many teenagers have begun to use computers as a substitute for interaction between themselves and other children of their own age group. They spend excessive time, surfing the web, talking in chat rooms, playing games, and thus they managed to spend their free time.

Such people are on their way to becoming incipient victims of future personality disorders. These people are addicted to their computers or to their cell phones. I know of a family, which sleeps with their own personal smart phones, right under their pillows. This is taking this obsession and addiction to a dangerous limit.

You may feel glad that you are doing something constructive on your computer. However, this screen time is interfering with your family, friends, work or school. Then you try cutting down this computer interaction time, you are going to feel anxious and irritable. Hey, you have not checked your mail during the last 15 minutes. You have not logged in on to your favorite social chat forum today. You have not found out what is up on your favorite site, and you are anxious to know whether anybody has responded to the note you wrote on it.

Does not this smack of possible incipient obsessive compulsive disorder? So if you find yourself interrupting your work in order to check your mail, make up a list.

This is what I told my friends to do. All of them are addicted to the screen. They are all suffering from this disorder which makes them log into chat rooms, email, and on the Internet to check up the status of what is happening where every 10 minutes.

I asked them to make a list of the time they check their email and to do it honestly. I also asked them to make a list of the time they logged on to their favorite websites just to browse, and the logging off time.

We pooled all the results together, just for fun, when we were relaxing over some fattening junk food, and to our horror, we were horrified at the result.

One of us had checked her smart phone for messages, 43 times in 5 ½ hours. One of us had logged in on to the Internet, to check email, 7 times in one hour.

In fact, we quite lost our appetites for chocolate éclairs and chicken mayonnaise burgers, when we saw this information, written by our own hands and written honestly, without skimping.

Is it a surprise that a number of us have subconsciously become so addicted to this activity, that we get irritated if we do not switch on the screen a number of times every day?

In fact, researchers have found a high degree of coordination between the time spent online, including chat rooms, and an increased incidence of depression.

This is a personality disorder which is going to increase as time goes by and our addiction/dependence on these gadgets is going to increase as time goes by, unless we discipline ourselves and learn how to monitor computer usage.

Is it any wonder why children are more sedentary than ever before? When once they spent their time outside, in the fresh air, running about and exercising their bodies, today they locked themselves up in a fuggy atmosphere of an ill aerated room, staring like zombies at a screen.

Their vocabulary consists of grunts in response to questions, because they are so busy beavering away on their computer screens/smart phones/tablets. For elementary school-age children, 4 – 5 hours in front of a computer screen is going to constitute an excessive amount of unconstructive time without any form of physical activity.

This is definitely detrimental to their physical health. So it is going to be the responsibility of a supervising adult, first of all to make sure that any child's activities on the computer is monitored with set times and limits for usage.

Children cannot afford a sedentary lifestyle during their growing stage, and neither can adults. So if you do not want to end up obese and overweight, remember that you are not a slave to your computer.

Myths about Computers and Children

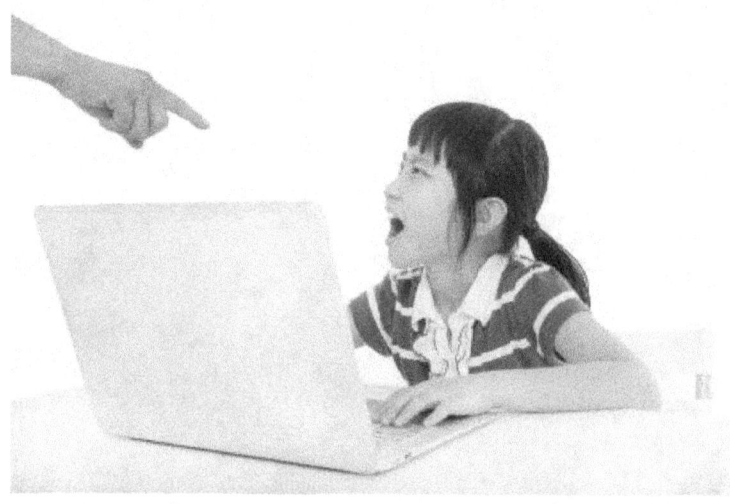

But Daaaaaad! My half hour on your laptop isn't up yet.

Here are some myths about computers, which have been explained and exploded.

Computers are not going to make your children smarter, even though many parents believe this. However, computers, software cannot teach your children concepts, which they are not ready for, developmentally.

Your computer should be considered just a supplement to increase knowledge, along with more concrete learning activities.

I remember my computer geek brother picking up his then 9-month-old baby boy and placing him on his lap. My brother was, at that time a computer addict and still is. But he wanted to spend some quality time with his little one. Even though his computer called him like a Lorelei.

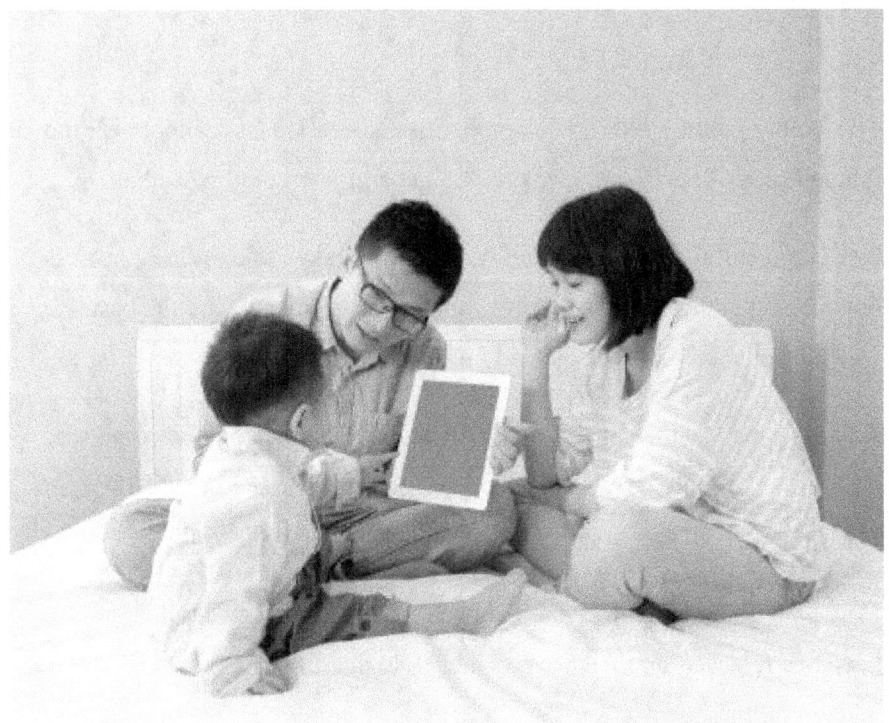

So he did something sensible. Knowing that it was not too early to begin teaching his baby about colors, he made sure that every day the display of the objects in the computer were in one particular color. So the child got to know about all the colors, at the age of 9 months.

He could point out the same color of an object on the table, with another object of that same color on the computer screen and I was really surprised to see this 9-month-old child showing his sense of achievement and happiness by chortling loudly, even though he communicated in inarticulate noises instead of words.

And naturally, he was really glad to have his papa kiss him and say well done, my sonny boy, whenever he made the correct choice, often 10 times out of 10, to our great amazement.

This young youth is extremely competitive today. He just cannot bear the thought of his best friend, managing to get a higher point in academics.

One could call this not very healthy, when it is taken to extremes, but this boy learned at the tender age of 9 months, that computers are the best way in which he can gain knowledge and polish up his skills.

And his papa is quite capable of ordering him to switch off the computer, if he goes one minute beyond the allocated computer usage time? How many of the parents out there really bother about such strict discipline?

Hey, I am going to answer that question, after I have checked this message, I have just received on my smart phone. Hold that thought.

So what was that question again?

There is another myth, which needs to be explained – sitting close to a computer screen is going to damage my child's eyes.

According to the American Academy of Ophthalmology, computer monitors are considered to be safe for normal use and do not present any hazard to the eyes through supposed emissions. However, you are going to suffer from eye strain, if you do not blink your eyes continuously.

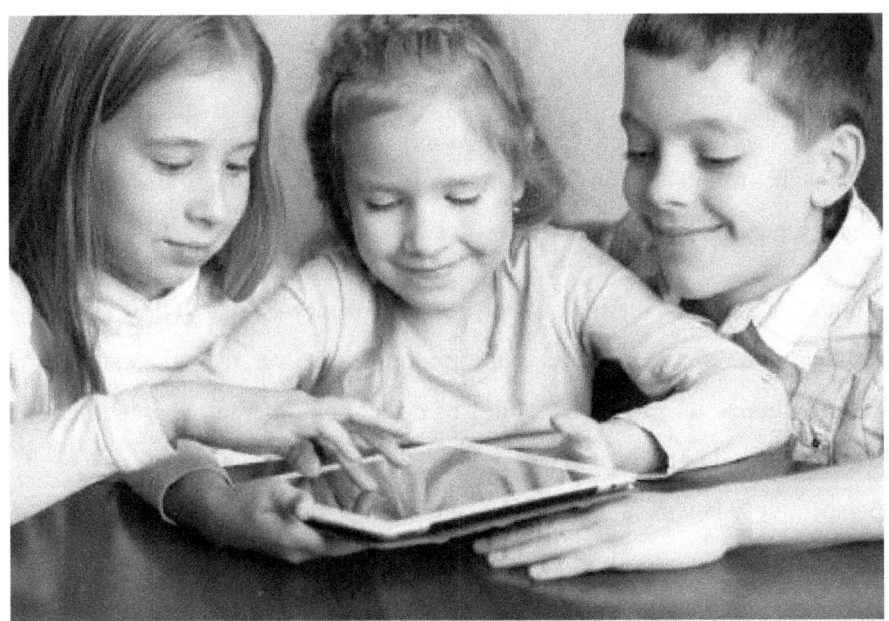

In the same way, computers do not give off harmful radiation. The electromagnetic rays which are given off by the computers are of the non-ionizing and safe variety. So you are not going to suffer from tumor, brain cancer, or any of those other scary diseases, which information has been given to you through the media, thanks to some statistics given out by some researchers.

I can assure you that those statistics are humbug and a possible leg pull by some malicious clowns.

As for the social aspect of excessive computer usage, naturally, you are going to be using your power of discipline, by restricting the computer usage within limits. That means your child is going to have plenty of time for socializing. But you will need to lead by example in such a case, and shut your smart phone/computer off.

Conclusion

So, where were we? I will be getting back to you, after I get up, stretch my legs, walk around a bit and twist my neck, back and forth and then get back to my screen ball and chain.

Computers, along with the Internet are quite phenomenal, and they can radically improve your access to information. However, as with nearly any benefit, there are some potential downsides of computer usage, which have been discussed in this book. Computers need to be put in their proper perspective. They should be used wisely in the context of your social and personal life as well as professional work commitments.

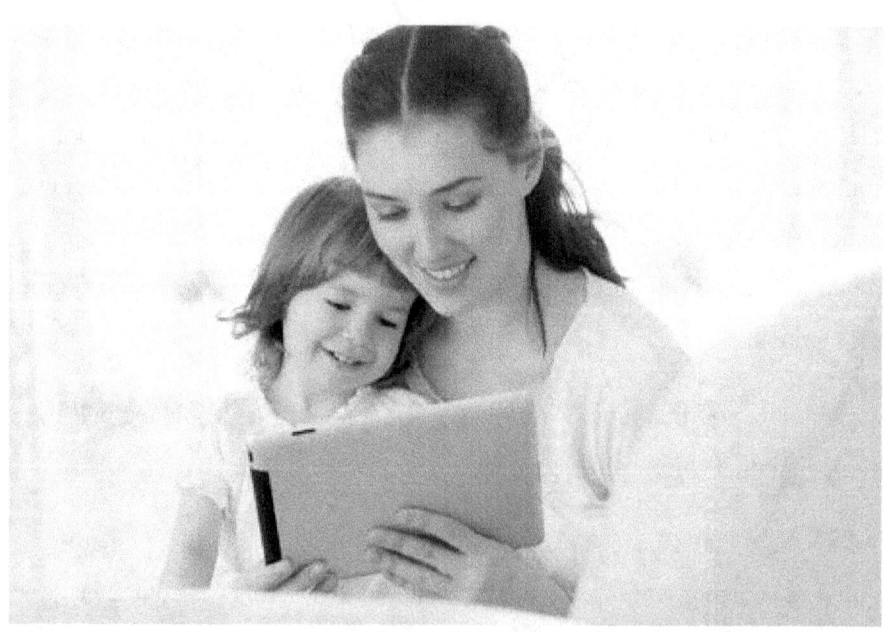

This book has also given you plenty of information on all the possible harmful effects prolonged computer usage could have upon your health. It also has tips and techniques, which are going to be useful to prevent RSI and carpal tunnel syndrome, which unfortunately is becoming more prevalent as more of us get addicted to computers.

So remember, your health is in your hands. A little bit of self-discipline today is going to prevent a lot of possible pain tomorrow. Also, just imagine if your hands are so painful that you could not use your computer and the doctor has strictly forbidden you to use it, until your muscles healed themselves?

What do you do under such circumstances? Do what I did, a couple of years ago, when shooting pains started in my wrist.

I got my priorities right. I needed to tackle this on the outset itself, because if it became nearly impossible for me to work on the computer due to pain, how would I earn my daily bread, butter and jam?

So I spent a month's leave in a remote place, where I had no access to computers or mice. That was after I told everybody that I was thinking of renouncing the world and they were not to bother me with official/personal/trivial worldly problems! They did not.

I spent my time in the open air, did plenty of outdoor work, and ate lots of healthy, nourishing food, like a hungry horse. Did wrist exercises in order to heal and rejuvenate the tissue. I also learned how to dance, with plenty of energetic wrist and hand movements.

When I came back home rejuvenated – and with hands and wrists healed –, the computer was not the be-all and end-all of my life. So be sensible, and decide that you are more important than a computer and ruining your health, through sheer inertia or apathy is not the act of a serious, mature and responsible person.

So, Live Long and Prosper, the Sensible Way.

Author Bio

Dueep Jyot Singh is a Management and IT Professional who managed to gather Postgraduate qualifications in Management and English and Degrees in Science, French and Education while pursuing different enjoyable career options like being an hospital administrator, IT,SEO and HRD Database Manager/ trainer, movie , radio and TV scriptwriter, theatre artiste and public speaker, lecturer in French, Marketing and Advertising, ex-Editor of Hearts On Fire (now known as Solstice) Books Missouri USA, advice columnist and cartoonist, publisher and Aviation School trainer, ex-moderator on Medico.in, banker, student councilor ,travelogue writer ... among other things!

One fine morning, she decided that she had enough of killing herself by Degrees and went back to her first love -- writing. It's more enjoyable! She already has 48 published academic and 14 fiction- in- different- genre books under her belt.

When she is not designing websites or making Graphic design illustrations for clients , she is browsing through old bookshops hunting for treasures, of which she has an enviable collection – including R.L. Stevenson, O.Henry, Dornford Yates, Maurice Walsh, De Maupassant, Victor Hugo, Sapper, C.N. Williamson, "Bartimeus" and the crown of her collection- Dickens "The Old Curiosity Shop," and "Martin Chuzzlewit" and so on… Just call her "Renaissance Woman") - collecting herbal remedies, acting like Universal Helping Hand/Agony Aunt, or escaping to her dear mountains for a bit of exploring, collecting herbs and plants and trekking.

Check out some of the other JD-Biz Publishing books

Gardening Series on Amazon

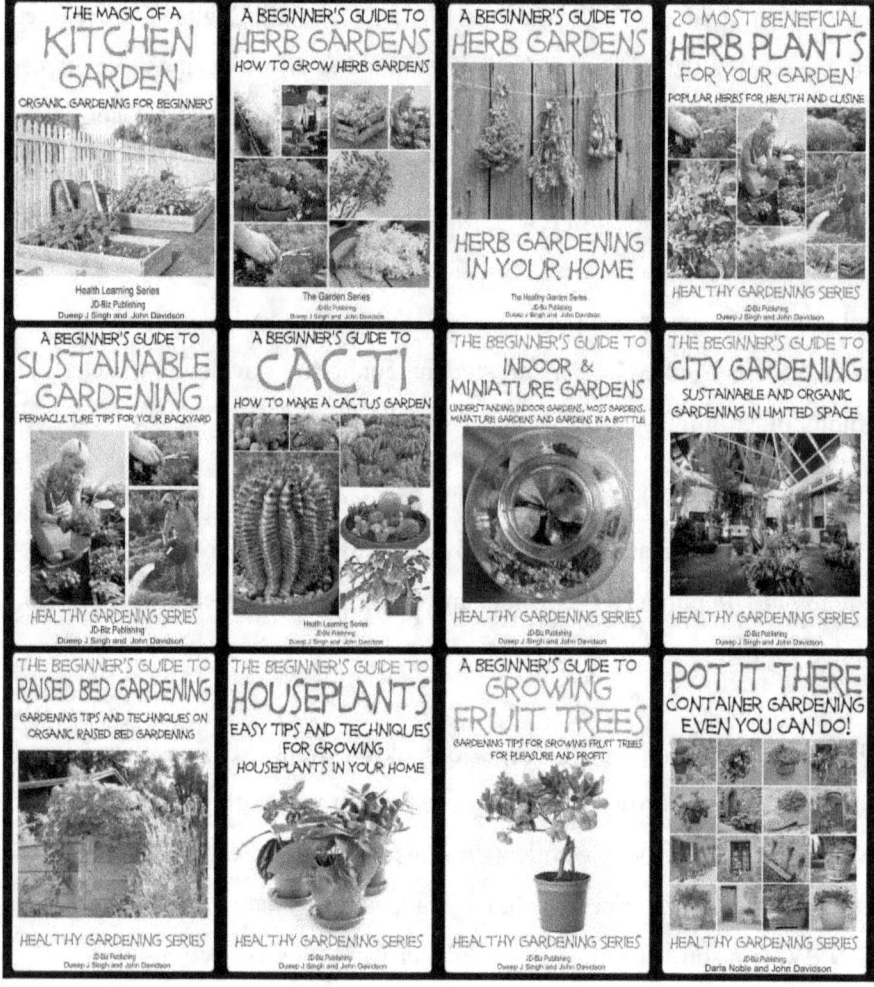

Health Learning Series

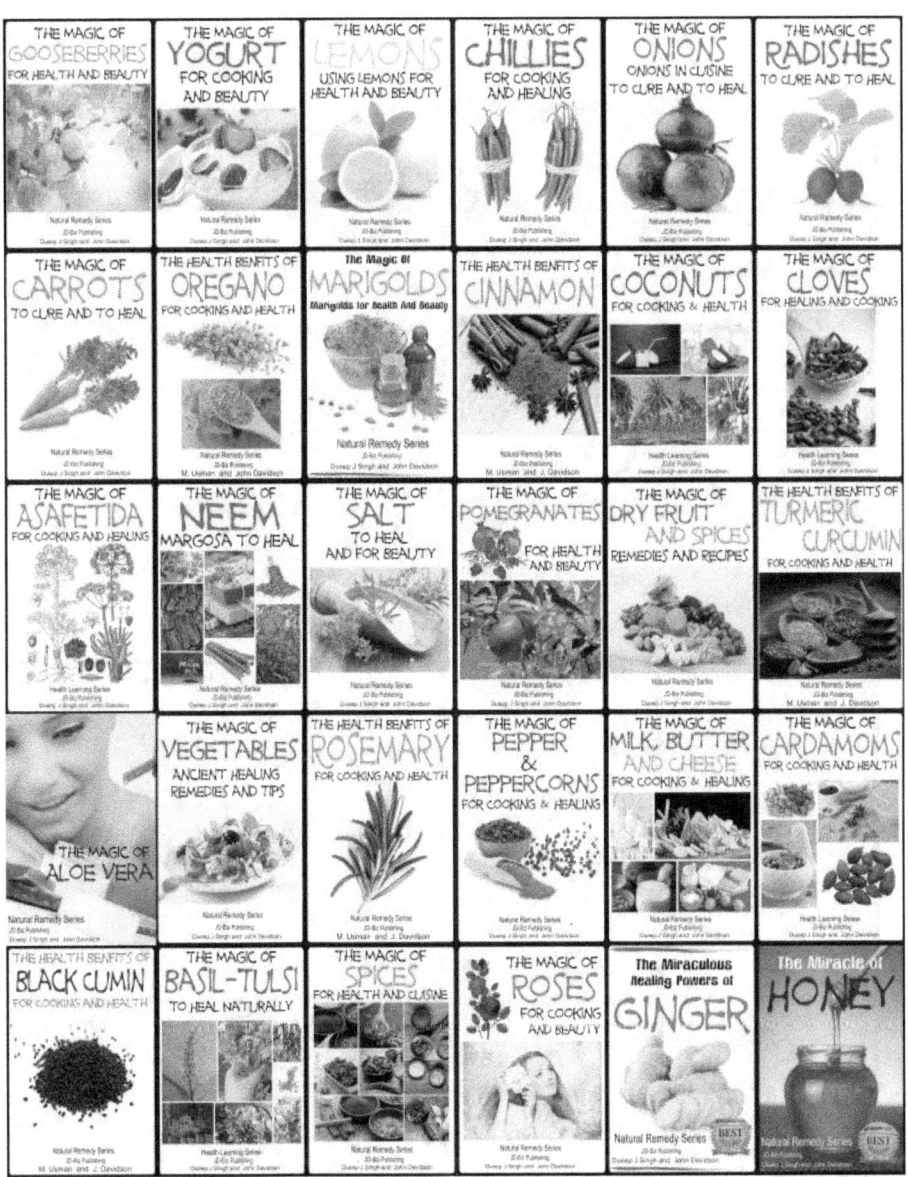

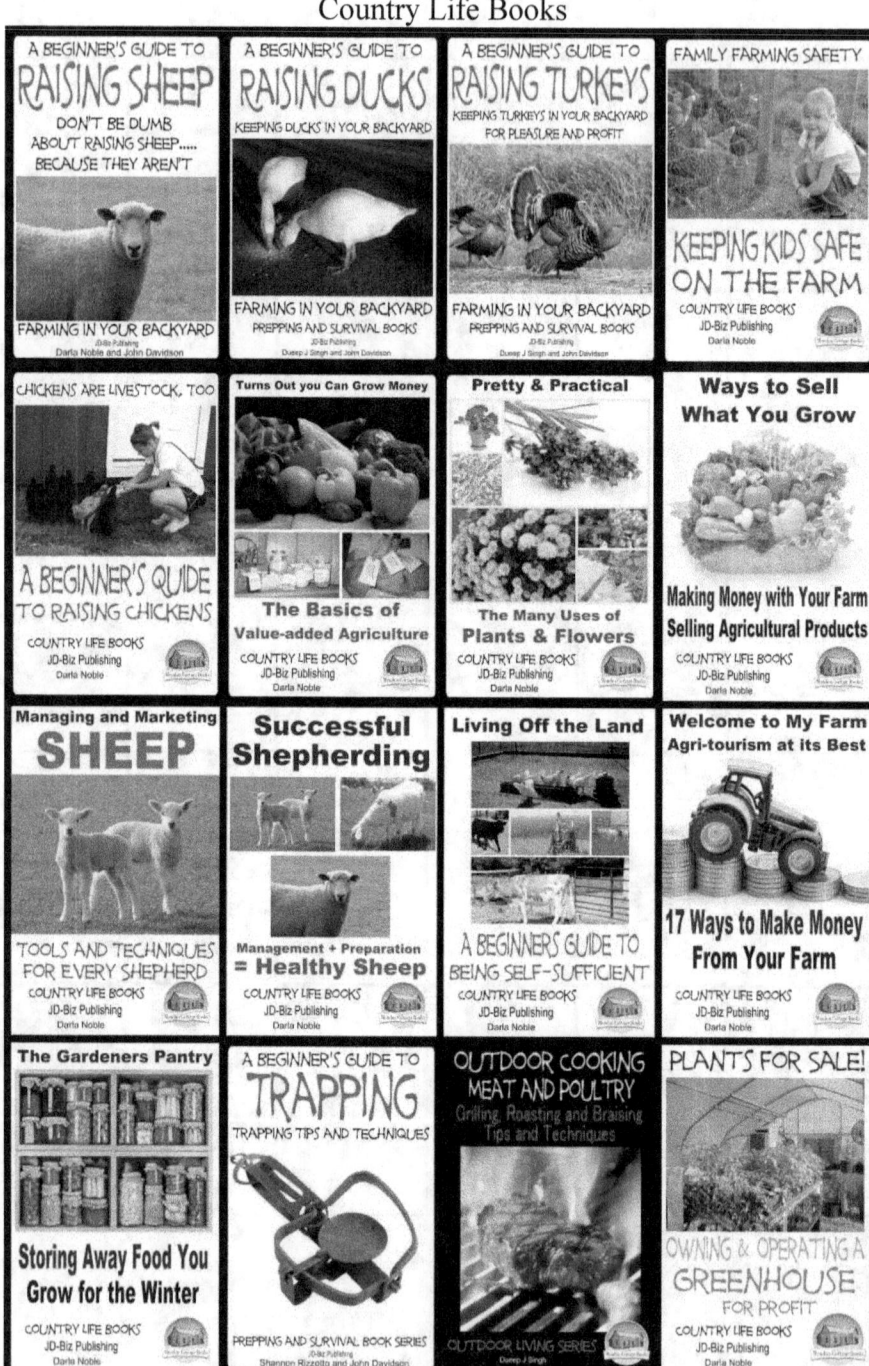

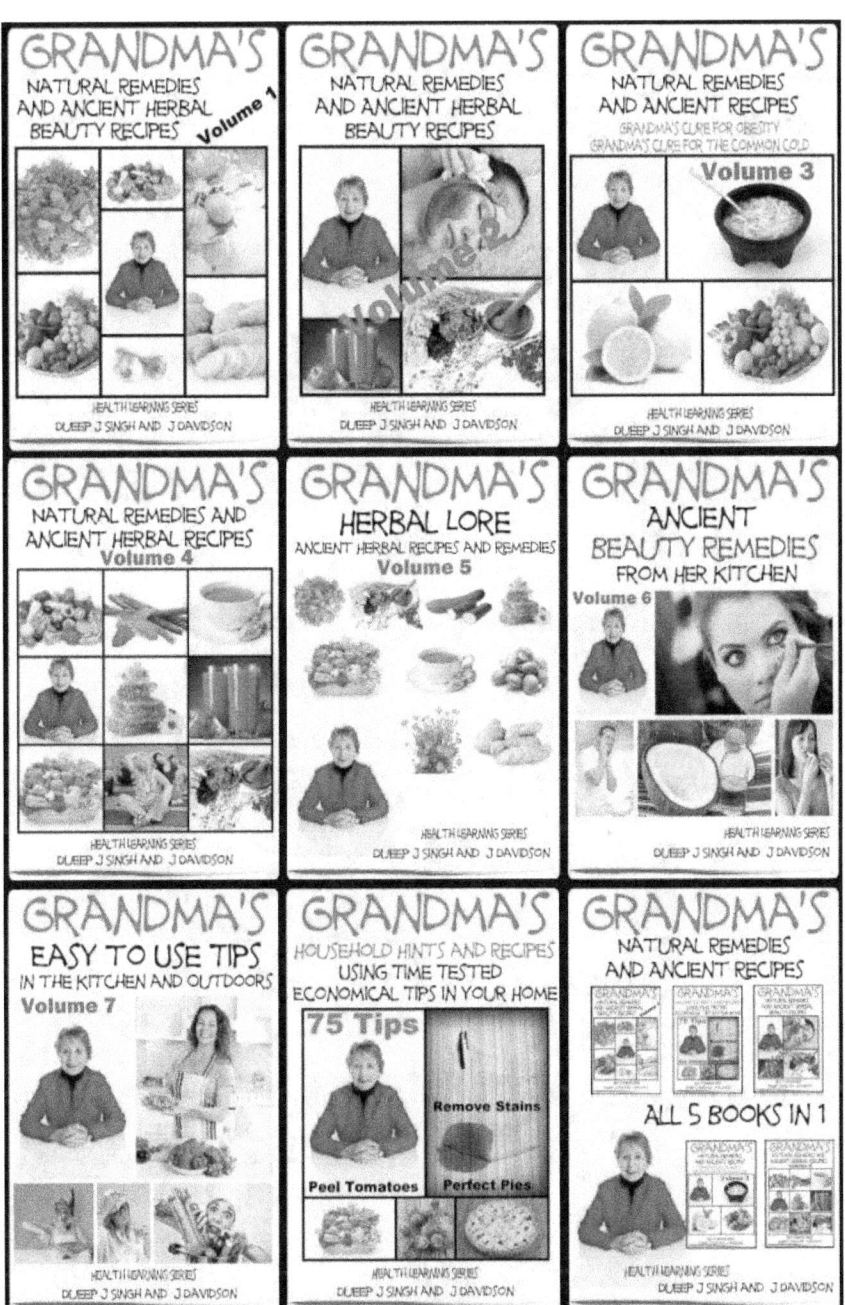

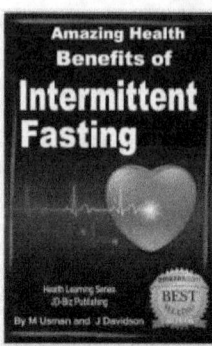

Amazing Health Benefits of Intermittent Fasting

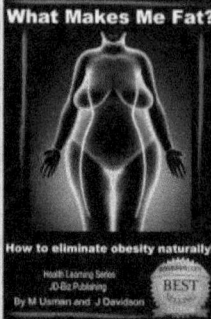

What Makes Me Fat?

How to eliminate obesity naturally!

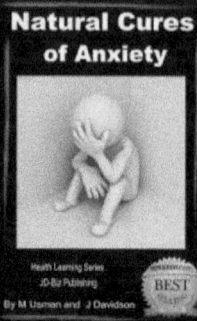

Natural Cures of Anxiety

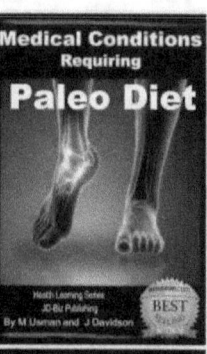

Medical Conditions Requiring Paleo Diet

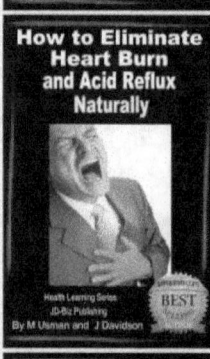

How to Eliminate Heart Burn and Acid Reflux Naturally

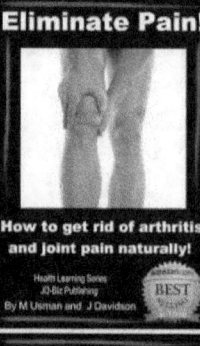

Eliminate Pain!

How to get rid of arthritis and joint pain naturally!

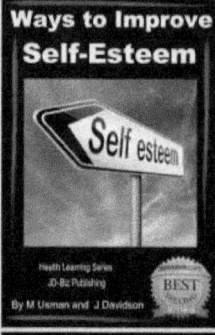

Ways to Improve Self-Esteem

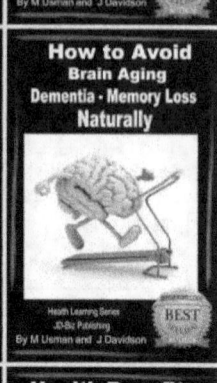

How to Avoid Brain Aging Dementia - Memory Loss Naturally

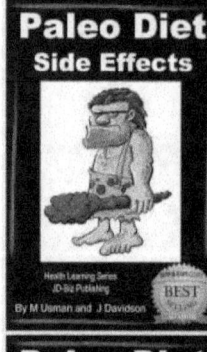

Paleo Diet Side Effects

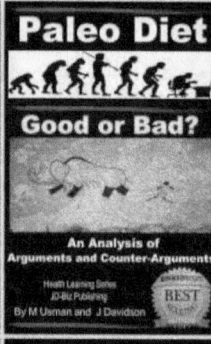

Paleo Diet Good or Bad?

An Analysis of Arguments and Counter-Arguments

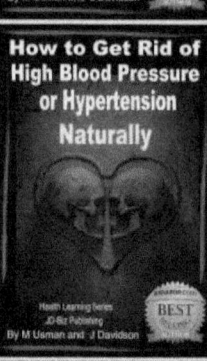

How to Get Rid of High Blood Pressure or Hypertension Naturally

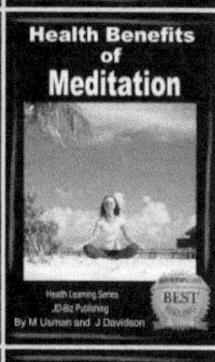

Health Benefits of Meditation

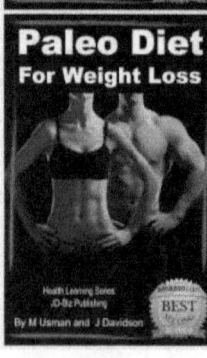

Paleo Diet For Weight Loss

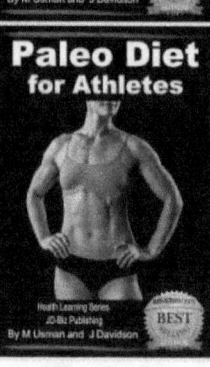

Paleo Diet for Athletes

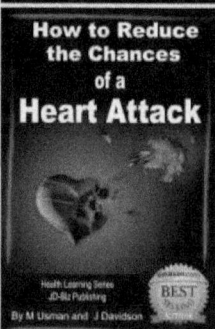

How to Reduce the Chances of a Heart Attack

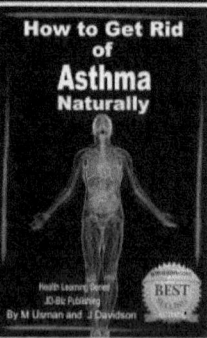

How to Get Rid of Asthma Naturally

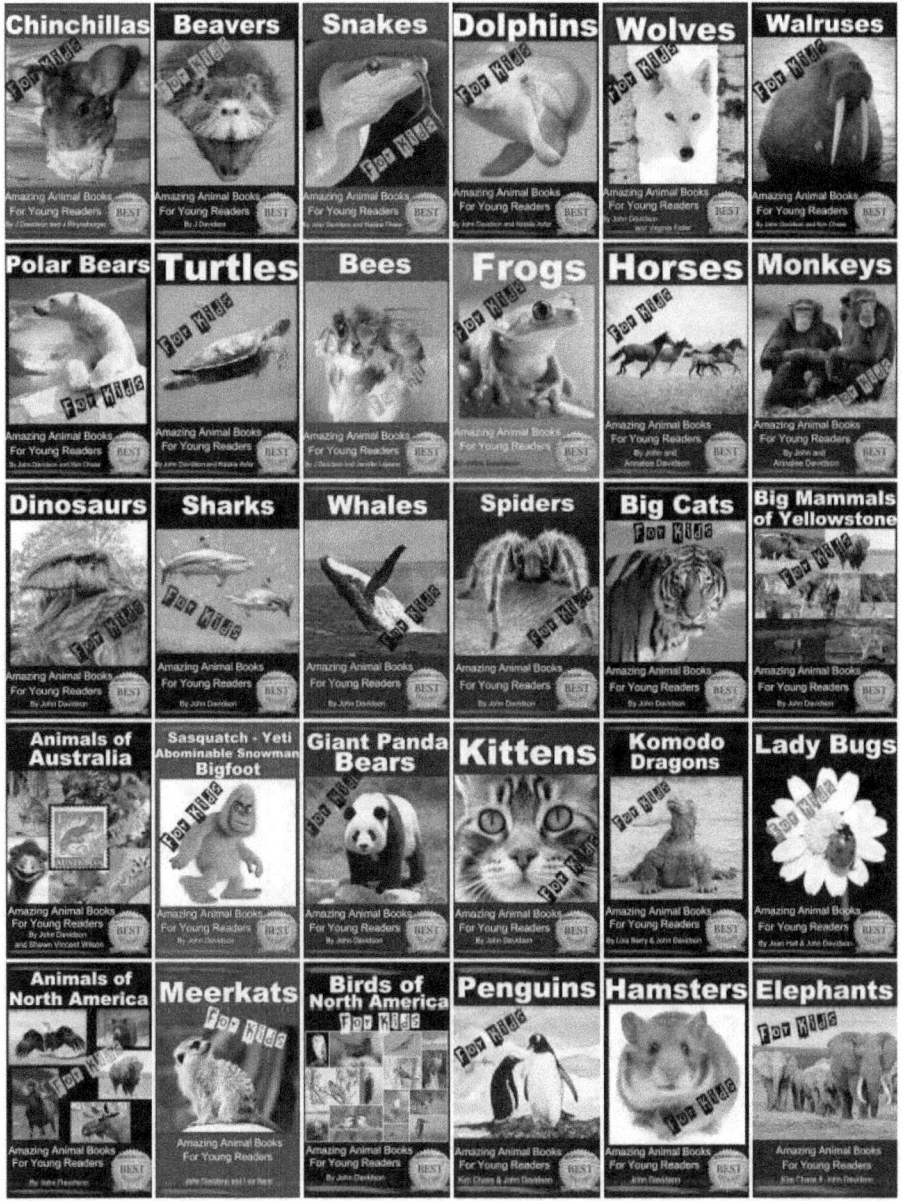

Learn To Draw Series

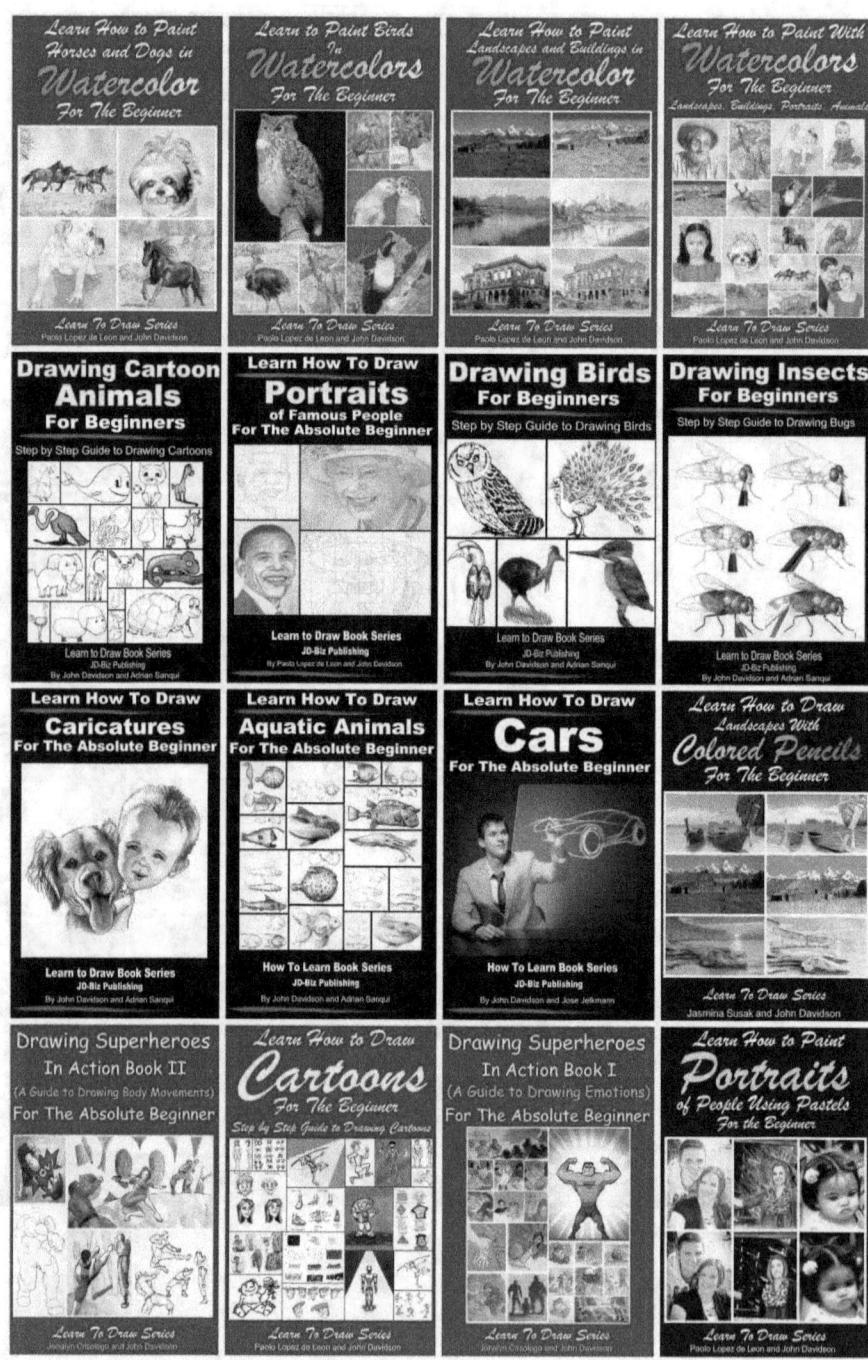

How to Build and Plan Books

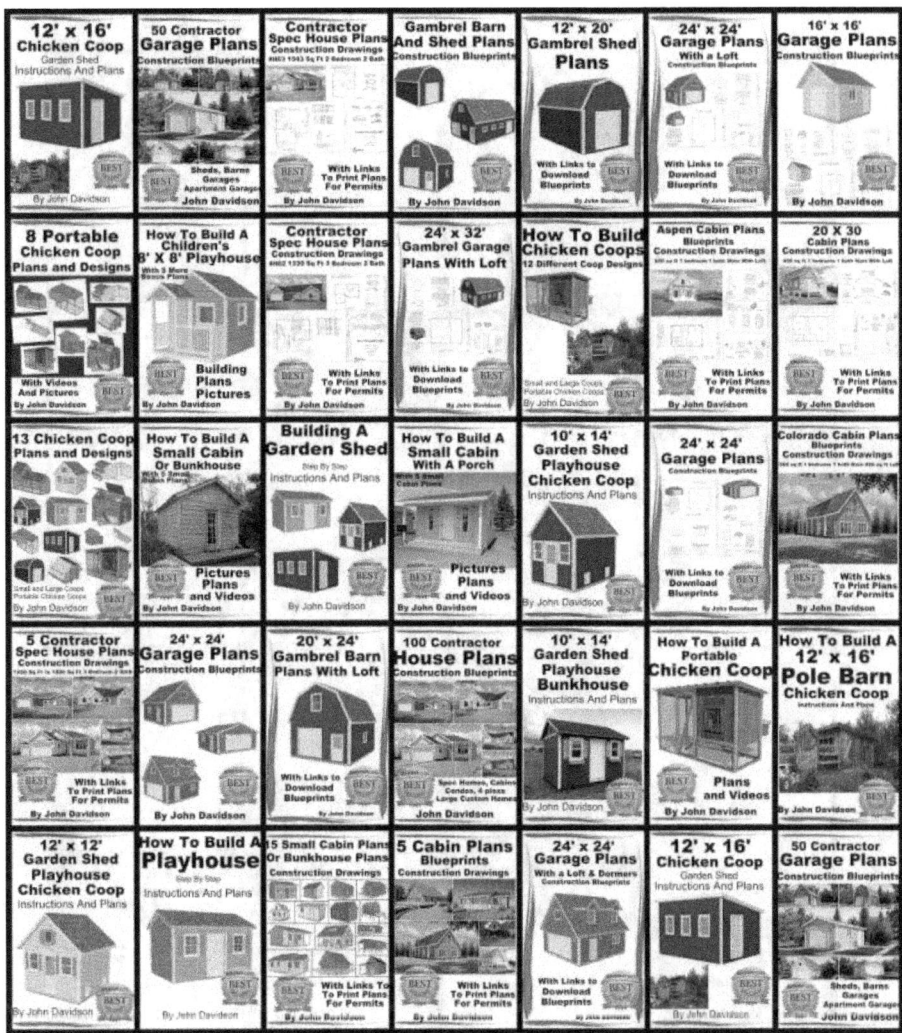

Entrepreneur Book Series

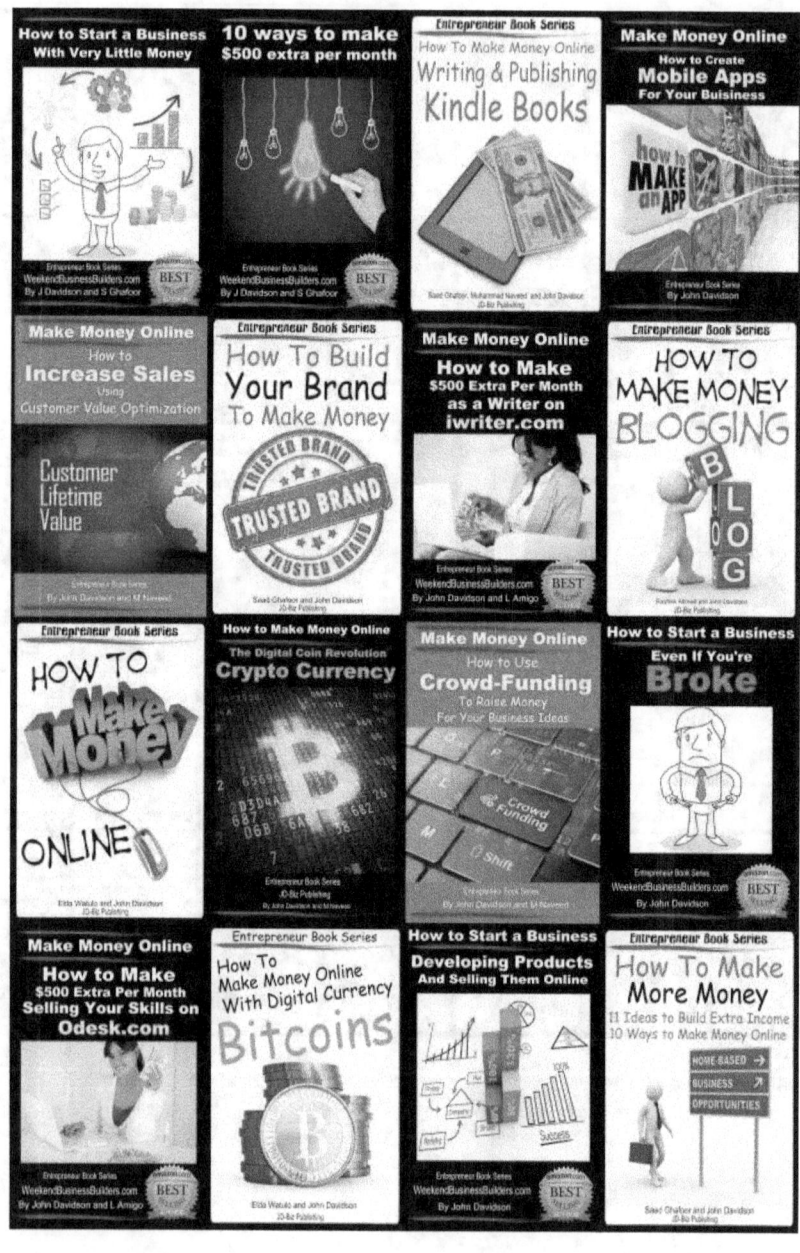

Our books are available at

1. Amazon.com

2. Barnes and Noble

3. Itunes

4. Kobo

5. Smashwords

6. Google Play Books

Publisher

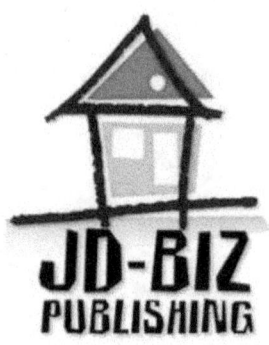

JD-Biz Corp

P O Box 374

Mendon, Utah 84325

http://www.jd-biz.com/

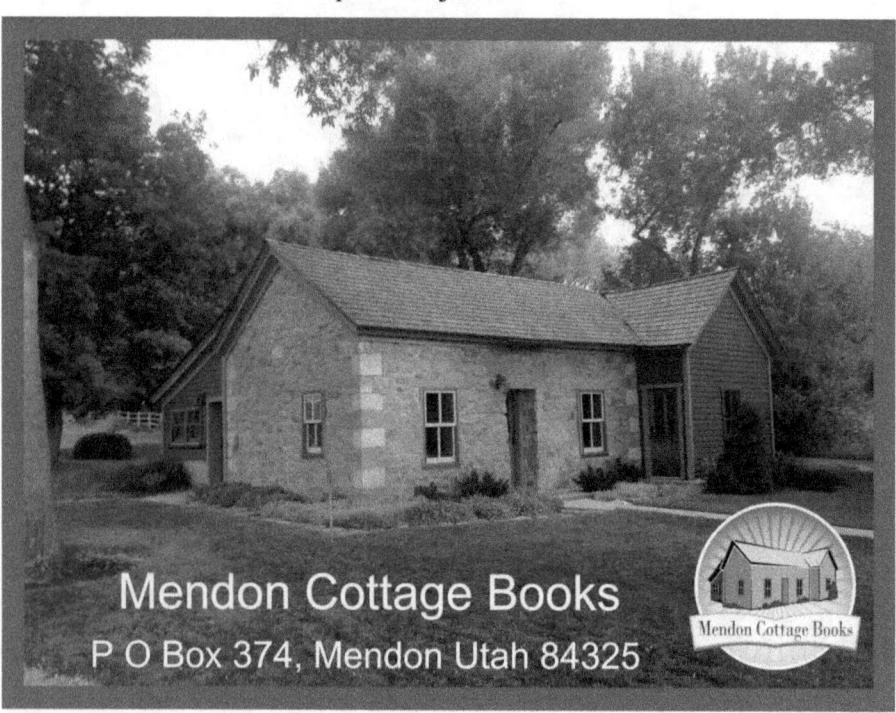

Mendon Cottage Books

P O Box 374, Mendon Utah 84325

www.ingramcontent.com/pod-product-compliance
Lightning Source LLC
Chambersburg PA
CBHW070332290526
45791CB00003B/1311